YOUR
DOCTOR CALLED
it's not time to retire

YOUR DOCTOR CALLED

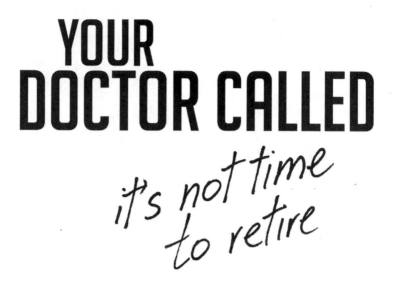

it's not time to retire

DAVID LEMON, MD

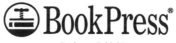
BookPress®

www.BookpressPublishing.com

Published in Des Moines, Iowa, by:

Bookpress Publishing
P.O. Box 71532, Des Moines, IA 50325
www.BookpressPublishing.com

Publisher's Cataloging-in-Publication Data

Names: Lemon, David K., author.
Title: Your Doctor Called – It's Not Time to Retire / David K. Lemon.
Description: Des Moines, IA: Bookpress Publishing, 2023.
Identifiers: LCCN: 2022920223 | ISBN: 978-1-947305-61-8
Subjects: LCSH Older people--Employment. | Retirement--Psychological aspects. | Retirement--Planning. | BISAC SELF-HELP / Aging | BUSINESS & ECONOMICS / Personal Finance / Retirement Planning
Classification: LCC HQ1062 .L46 2023| DDC 646.79--dc23

First Edition
Printed in the United States of America
10 9 8 7 6 5 4 3 2 1

This book is dedicated to my wife Suzanne.

It is also dedicated to my parents,

Ken and Marge Lemon,

who tragically died in an airplane crash,

leaving my life all too early.

CONTENTS

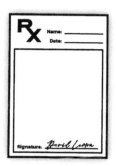

Prologue

"Hello, Mr. (or Ms.) 'Smith!' I'm glad to meet you. I'm Dr. Lemon. How may I help you?"

Over the past fifty years, I've had the privilege of asking that question again and again. I am a physician practicing cardiology in central Iowa. It has been a very meaningful and eventful journey to care for others who put their trust in me to make the most appropriate decisions about their hearts and their health. As the years have gone by, I now realize that I am nearing the end of that journey.

Generally, as Americans, we are privileged to be able to make retirement decisions. As I write this book, reflecting on my own thoughts and ideas about slowing down and retirement, my purpose is to share the wisdom I've gained through my patients' views of their retirement journeys.

People who have worked their entire lives view retirement from many perspectives. Some anxiously cannot wait to retire, while others fear not having to set the alarm or not having to check in at a certain time. The idea brings a host of emotional, financial, and lifestyle concerns. Some greatly anticipate finally having time to do things they have always wanted to do—play more golf, travel with a spouse, and spend more time with grandkids. Some are anxious about the end of a career, fear they'll outlive their finances, or simply don't know what to do next. No matter the path people choose, critical decisions bring a great deal of stress. Considerations include financial issues as well as possible changes in relationships, housing, healthcare needs, and just what to do with all that newly found time.

My mindset over the years has been to do the work, stay educated and up-to-date in my field, and to do the right thing for my patients. The idea and uncertainty of retirement are intimidating to me, but I am not alone. Perhaps the insight my patients have given me can help us all work our way to good decisions for ourselves, our families, our colleagues, and all those in our lives.

I would like to acknowledge and thank the many patients I interviewed who openly shared their best wit, wisdom, and insights on retirement. Their candid and honest responses are greatly appreciated. Of course, their names are changed to protect their privacy.

I would also like to thank my wife, Suzanne, for her assistance in writing and editing.

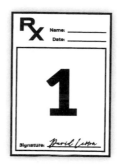

A Brief History of the
Concept of Retirement

Before the modern age, the idea of retirement was irrelevant. People worked until they died or until they could no longer work due to old age or infirmity. Many years ago, when the average life expectancy was age 40, a person's daily existence consisted of hard work and the hope that they would not succumb to illness or injury. The future was about tomorrow, literally. As life expectancy increased along with the advent of the industrial revolution, the idea of retirement came into focus.

In 1881, Otto von Bismarck, the German chancellor, presented a radical idea to the Reichstag: government-run financial support for older members of society—retirement. By the end of the decade, the German government would create a retirement system for citizens over the age of 70—if they lived that long. That retirement age aligned with the upper edge of life expectancy in Germany at the time. Even with retirement, most people still worked until they died.[1]

Military pensions originated in ancient Rome for soldiers who had risked their lives, although those pensions didn't necessarily mean they could stop working altogether. In the United States, starting in the mid-1800s, certain municipal employees—firefighters, police officers, and teachers—began receiving public pensions, primarily in large cities. In 1875, the American Express Company started offering private pensions.[2]

Around the world today, people in different countries view retirement differently. In Japan, the population is among the oldest on the planet. They're considering raising the retirement age to 70-75 to ease pension burdens and a labor crunch.[3] In France, the retirement age is 62.[4]

In the 20th century in the United States, the Great Depression and World War II radically changed ideas about life. Medical discoveries and the introduction of antibiotics and vaccines helped to increase the average life span. The Social Security Act was signed into law in 1935 and provided a guaranteed income to retired workers aged 65 and older. Public and private pensions and additional income from Social Security made retirement possible for older workers. The advent of Medicare in 1965 brought access and the availability of improved medical care to all who qualified, resulting in the average life span continuing to grow over the next several decades.

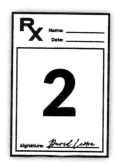

Effects of Coronavirus on Retirement Decisions

Baby Boomers, born between 1946 and 1964,[5] began reaching retirement age in 2011 and since 2015, represent 45% of the United States population.[6] In 2019-2020, however, the Covid-19 pandemic began giving all of us a new perspective on work, retirement, leisure, and a re-evaluation of what we thought was important. Before the pandemic and the lockdowns, how often did we lament, "If only I had more time. I'm tired of work. I want to go home,"? Well, that's where we found ourselves. Then we said, "If only I could go to work. I want to be productive."

Online media is helpful for remote work, but it's not the real thing. Most prefer to interact with real people face to face, make in-person decisions, and have our voices heard by real people. Some are now back to working in person again, while others continue to work remotely from home or are not working at all. In early 2022, thousands of companies that had closed their offices to in-person working two years ago have still not announced plans to return. On average, only 33% of the workforce has returned to the office.[7]

The unstructured nature of retirement might be a little like the pandemic. Those working remotely during the pandemic found themselves in uncharted waters as they navigated the balance between the demands of jobs and the needs and distractions of family and home. Those who thrived on inter-actions and relationships with co-workers found themselves without those supportive and encouraging people. Those who lost jobs found isolation and lack of financial earnings very difficult.

Alcohol consumption spiked during the pandemic.[8] Some of those who retired also found the adjustment quite difficult and resorted to increased alcohol consumption and some-times alcohol abuse.[9]

Until 2019, Baby Boomers had begun retiring at a pace of about two million a year, a rate of 1.5%. The Covid-19 pandemic, however, vastly changed the landscape for older Americans. Many people began retiring early, while some postponed retirement, the direct result of the pandemic. In the third quarter of 2019, 25.4 million Boomers were retired. In the same quarter of 2020, about 3.3 million more retired, shooting up to 3.2%. From February to November 2020 alone, the number of retiring Boomers increased by 1.1 million.

More than half the estimated 5.25 million people who left the workforce during the Covid-19 pandemic appear to have retired earlier than planned for several reasons. Being more vulnerable to serious infection, some older workers were inclined to stay away from jobs requiring a physical presence. Others found greater wealth in the sharp increase in stock prices and real estate values. Still, many others in various industries were laid off and retired not by choice. Some of those close to the traditional retirement age of 65 remain out of the workforce today.[10] Many feel that some of these temporarily retired workers will re-enter the labor force when the pandemic subsides. However, some economists expect that a high proportion of these jobs are lost for good.[11]

Some of those who have postponed retirement have found working remotely to be an asset. Working from home, they no longer must deal with grueling commutes or the stresses and potential health risks of being in an office.[12] A report found that two-thirds of people who have delayed retirement have done so because of Covid-19.[13]

In mid-2022, inflation hit 9.1%, forcing many to reconsider retirement. Others are leaving their previous retirement to go back to work.

According to CNBC, "Americans' finances are being squeezed as inflation pushes up prices on things such as rent, groceries, and gasoline. As a result, one-quarter of Americans will have to delay their retirement, according to the BMO Real Financial Progress Index, a quarterly survey conducted between March 30 and April 25, 2022. Putting off retirement plans is mostly due to disrupted savings from increased prices, the survey found. Thirty-six percent of survey respondents have reduced their savings, and 21% are putting away less for retirement to keep up with growing costs."[14]

Where Are We Now?

When I began studying and practicing medicine around 1970, the average life expectancy was 70. Over the years, sanitation has continued to improve, people are exercising for better health, and medical care continues to improve. Life-extending procedures like coronary artery bypass surgery, stents, and other procedures have evolved, rapidly improved, and become the standard of care.

According to PubMed.gov, "Ischemic heart disease (IHD) persists as the leading cause of death in the Western world. In recent decades, great headway has been made in reducing mortality due to IHD, based around secondary prevention. The advent of coronary revascularization techniques, first coronary artery bypass grafting surgery in the 1960s and then percutaneous coronary intervention (PCI) in the 1970s, has represented one of the major breakthroughs in medicine during the last century. The benefit provided by these techniques, especially PCI, has been crucial in lowering mortality rates in acute coronary syndrome."[15]

Advances in cancer care and exercise have also extended lives. One Harvard study found that "highly active men are 47% less likely to develop [colon cancer] than their sedentary peers."[16]

Over the last 50 years in the United States, lifespan has continued to increase. Women can now, on average, expect to live well into their 80s, and men are not far behind. However, life expectancy declined by a year and a half in 2020. Covid-19 deaths represented 74% of the decline.[17] Other causes of death surrounding Covid-19 included increased drug abuse deaths and the number of suicides, likely associated with isolation and depression. In a COVID-19 special report in *Hopkins Bloomberg*, "Experts warn that secondary effects of the pandemic and strategies to mitigate it could spark an uptick in suicides in the U.S., accelerating a trend that's been growing over the past two decades."[18]

However, with the general increase in longevity, new and unique problems have appeared. We may find ourselves alone and asking, "What am I supposed to do at age 82?"

Even with exceptional medical care, a great attitude, and exercise, the body and, to some extent, the mind "wear out." Friends may not be around. Family may be scattered all over the country. Many previously irrelevant questions now enter the picture with no sure answers.

Will I run out of money?

Am I a nuisance to my family?

What if I slip and fall?

Can I renew my driver's license?

Can I go to church?

Should I volunteer?

Do they want an old fogey around?

Then the questions and concerns about tomorrow start to become real.

What am I supposed to do now?

I feel isolated.

I want to be worthwhile.

I really don't want to go to a nursing home and be just another old person.

Maybe I'll make an appointment to see my doctor or preacher; they can help.

I need to write down a plan. Doesn't retire really mean 're-tire'?

The questions and concerns flood our minds.

Why should I take medications? I've already proven I don't need medicines to live long.

Why diet? Who cares if I'm overweight or underweight?

I've always been a rebel. Maybe I just won't take my medicines.

I'll just eat what I want.

But then, I really do want to see my grandkids grow up.

*I do enjoy talking to the guy at the coffee shop
(even if I can't remember his name).*

*I want the good old days. Wait a second, were they really
any better than today? Romanticizing the past only
makes the present feel worse.*

*I hate that cellphone. What is my password? Why do we
need a password for everything?*

We will all go through variations on this theme as we grow
older. Retirement without a plan for what to do next leads to
depression, frailty, and uncertain financial situations, among
other things. If you add isolation and health issues, the need
for a walker, memory problems, and the inability to drive, it
soon leads to despair.

For some, retirement is actually worse for their health than
for those who continue working. A study by the Harvard
School of Public Health was revealing. They looked at rates
of heart attack and stroke among men and women in the
ongoing U.S. Health and Retirement Study.[19] Among 5,422
individuals in the study, those who had retired were 40% more
likely to have had a heart attack or stroke than those who were
still working. The increase was more pronounced during the
first year after retirement and leveled off after that.[20]

We "young" oldsters who continue to work and don't want
to retire are always looking over our shoulders to see if the
young bucks are laughing at us.

Constantly the boss wants us to be productive.

Can I do it? I want to, but am I able?

They don't ask my opinions anymore. I'm not part of "future planning."

But life can be good. Work can be rewarding. Slow down. Talk to people and listen. Appreciate the simple things; appreciate the routine.

Maybe it's ok to wear out. Better than to 'rust out.'

It's ok to take a nap on Saturday; on Monday I'll be ready to go.

Speak up and tell them: Here is my opinion.

I want to bring home the bacon.

I want to live long, die quickly, and not be a burden.

Work often defines men more than women, and it defines me. I'm not ashamed to admit that fact. Work like it's God's work and His plan for you and me, because it is. Most of us have worked all our lives, and right or wrong, it defines our worth. The very rich probably can't relate to this. As I watch television, advertisements and programming are not aimed at me. *Maybe I need to take a walk and unwind.*

As I write this, we are now well into the coronavirus pandemic and hopefully getting past the worst of it. People are tired of the many previous restrictions, lockdowns, mandates, and masks. Vaccines are readily available. The virus seems as if it's here to stay and may be getting less virulent. Many people are still working from home, the economy is up and down, and the 'experts' still don't know how to overcome all this. As their sometimes-conflicting directives prevailed, many people lost trust in medical experts, politicians, government, media, and public health institutions.

I want to leave you with a quote from an article entitled, *The Collapse of Trust in Public Health*. "There is a potential social cost to this loss in trust. Public health in the last century largely did good for humanity, with its emphasis on holistic perspectives on human well-being, the distribution of therapeutics and vaccines, the education on clean water and wise disease mitigation, its focus on rational science and calm over disease panic, and so much more. With lockdowns, and the tremendous public confusion sown by so many, this entire well-deserved reputation for science in the public interest is in tatters."[21]

Restoration of trust in public health and other institutions will be slow to return.

What the Real Experts Have to Say

Women and men often see work and retirement differently. Women can multitask better than men, often are more adaptable to change, and have a wider network of friends, family, and social contacts. A TIAA survey found that retired women are more likely than men to be busy caregiving, socializing with friends and family, and giving back to the community; retired men are more likely to be engaged in sports and working.[22]

The people I interviewed for this book are my patients. I see them in my daily work as a physician. The following are some of their views and comments about work and retirement. I think their wit and wisdom are not only amusing but may open our eyes to some truths.

Marie has been my patient for some time. She is 75 years old. She has been retired from her "not at home" job for 15 years. She tells me she has never been so busy. She volunteers whenever and wherever the chance arises. She wants to be helpful. She is a quilter and loves to make things for family and friends. She is bright and cheery and is always positive and adapts. Her husband is a farmer, or more accurately, "was" a farmer. He told me he was afraid that he would "lose his identity" and wouldn't be able to tell himself and others who he was because he felt that who he was seemed to be defined by what he did—farming. His solution was to find a "new" job. Now he does woodworking, and he loves it. It calms him down and gives him purpose. They didn't retire; they just changed jobs.

The message is clear. We need to work in one way or another. We need to be relevant, and work of some sort fills that need. It doesn't have to be a structured job with pay. Women seem to adapt better to retirement than men because they usually were the primary caregivers as they raised a family. Their role changed as the children aged, and they rolled along with the change as well. Sometimes, as men, we have "forever" jobs, or careers, with less change and more structure. That's great when you are young, but as we near retirement age, not so good.

Harold is 82 years old. He is a doctor. He told me that he makes a new "Five-Year Plan" every five years. He started doing that at age 60. He says he will keep working until he can't do it anymore. He looks at his life in an organized, updated assessment and then just does it. Having a plan appears to be the key. He is always thinking about what's next, not about yesterday. A plan means he is optimistic about tomorrow and wants to be prepared. Might it mean he is a guy who likes to control things? Probably. It also sounds like someone who doesn't want to sit around and coast through the last years of life. If you're good at what you do and you enjoy it, why would you quit doing it?

Edward is my neighbor. I see him frequently when I take a walk around the neighborhood. He is always friendly and has a great smile. He is about 75 years old. He retired about six years ago, but got bored. To remedy his boredom, he now wakes up at three every morning. He eats breakfast and then heads off to Menard's, where he stocks shelves from five to nine every morning, six days a week. He tells me if he works 1,000 hours per year, they will give him a bonus. He works out every day. He is very physically fit. He always has a nice word to say about someone or some situation. He says he still climbs ladders and takes care of his yard—and it looks beautiful. Edward is too busy to get old. He has a great attitude, and every day is full of worthwhile, meaningful activities. He looks forward to each day. He doesn't complain or focus on what he doesn't have or might need. I'll admit, Edward is a great role model, and is who we all would like to imitate. Do more. Keep busy. Keep a routine. Stay involved. It's been said, "Your attitude about who you are and what you have is a very little thing that makes a very big difference."[23]

Another patient, **Jeannie**, told me, "I hated retiring. I was a teacher, and I grieved for a whole year. But my daughter said she had hit the jackpot. I now help take care of her six kids."

In retirement, she had lost her sense of worth and reason for getting up each morning. Every day while teaching, she gave of herself; she had a purpose, discipline, and the joy of seeing her work in her students' achievements and gratitude. Then it was gone. Why get up in the morning? Who cares what I do? No lesson plans to make, no meetings to attend, no agenda, no deadlines. At the time, she probably bemoaned the schedule and discipline, but later realized it defined who she was and why she got up each day. But now she's back. Six kids, discipline, chaos. She can teach and fret and worry over her grandkids. She can get tired. Life is good and has meaning for her once again.

Bernice is a very elderly lady with a fighting spirit. When I asked her about retirement and what it meant to her, I was blown away by her ability to determine what really matters. She told me, "I can't see, I can't hear, but I can still talk. I still know a little."

She tells us a lot about getting old and fighting the feeling of irrelevance and being forgotten. Maybe her eyes and ears don't work very well anymore, but "she" is still here in many ways. She still has an important voice that deserves to be heard. She has lifelong wisdom, she can still contribute, and we ought to listen up. Like Bernice, we may not be what we used to be, but we can still be relevant because we, too, "know a little."

Jeanette is 68 years old. She has lung cancer and has had a coronary artery bypass operation. She still works full-time! I asked her what advantage she might have if she retired. With a wry laugh, she said, "I wouldn't feel so rushed."

When I think about it, she is saying, "If I work hard and feel rushed, I won't sit and mope and worry about my lung cancer and my bad heart." If we are mentally and physically busy, we don't sit around and worry about tomorrow and don't dwell on bad things from our past. Too much time to think can be a dangerous thing. Too many options increase our anxiety. Life is hard enough, but if we have purpose and a job, we can focus on today, not on tomorrow or yesterday. It's easy to say but hard to do. But having a job, a purpose, and a plan for today decreases anxiety and helps us live in the present.

Tom, age 76, grinned and told me, "Doc says I'm living on borrowed time. I told him I want to borrow as much as I can." Tom may be getting old, but he still loves life and wants as much of it as he can get.

Ned gave some good advice. "Treat your body like a temple, not an amusement park." His advice is so true. As we age, we must take care of our bodies and minds. Don't do unwise things or take unnecessary risks.

"As we grow older, many changes occur within us both physically and emotionally, and it can be stressful to cope with the aging process. The vitality we once had as young men and women is now gone. Indeed, even though people generally enjoy a longer life expectancy nowadays, the aging process can be a painful fact to come to terms with."[24] Heart health, bone health, brain and nervous system health, and all body systems are impacted by advancing age.

Richard is a finance guy with his own business and is still working. I've known Richard for many years. He always has a smile and something clever to say. Richard says he is never going to retire. "Why?" I ask him. With a wide grin, he quips, "It's like this. If I don't like a client, I just don't schedule a return visit, or I give them to one of my partners." He is very organized, knows his business well, and how to make his work as enjoyable and rewarding as possible. He also walks three miles every day. It's half a mile to the track and half a mile back home. He walks around the track first in lane eight, then lane seven, and so forth until he walks around in lane one, making his measured three miles.

"Heart disease is the leading killer of American men. Because exercise helps improve so many cardiac risk factors (cholesterol, blood pressure, diabetes, obesity, and stress), it should have a powerful protective influence on heart attacks —and it does." Back in 1978, the Harvard Alumni Study found that men who exercise regularly are 39% less likely to suffer heart attacks than their sedentary peers. It was a ground-breaking observation, and it's been confirmed many times over.[25]

Richard's approach to life has a lot we can take to heart. If he doesn't like a client or situation and can't work in it, he walks away or laterals to a partner. Let's face it, there are people or situations we don't like and can't change or control. Sometimes running away from situations in life means retiring from work. That's a sad reality that hastens retirement for a lot of people. Perhaps a better alternative might be finding a new gig, working in a different office, or having a heart-to-heart talk with the offender. It's often challenging, but in the long run, it may lead to a better day-to-day approach to keep working.

Louise is 86 years young. When I asked her about the idea of retirement or slowing down, she told me, "You lose ground if you sit around." That mindset has evidently worked for her! "Sitting around" is passive. It weakens the body, elevates blood pressure, and leads to obesity. It also leads to boredom, pessimism, and constant complaints about the state of the world. When they do get up after sitting around, they're short of breath and dizzy, so they sit around some more. It's a downward spiral that unnecessarily impacts mental and physical health in negative ways.

Some patients quipped about how they manage retirement, the aches and pains of aging, and the reality of their mortality.

One patient, **Steve**, told me, "I know how you can get rid of pain." I asked how. "Die," he said. He's a kidder, but he's right. We all will likely have aches and pain and probably more of them as we age.

Fred told me, "My wife put a phone number on my running shoes. It was to Dunn's Funeral Home."

George said, "The main problem with death is that it is permanent."

Mike laughed and said, "I read the obituaries every day to see if my name is in there." Mike has the same idea as George. Don't dwell on death—we may as well make light of it as long as we can.

Bruce told me, "The more you do, the more you can do." He is 82.

Bruce should be a cardiologist. I tell my patients the same thing.

These men are all convinced that daily exercise along with

good nutrition and a good attitude are the most important components of maintaining health in advancing age.

Genevieve works at John Deere. She told me, "I see all these women retire. Then I read in the paper they died two years later. Nothing to do."

Here we go again. We wait eagerly to retire, but then what? Unfortunately, many don't have a plan. Emotionally they felt retirement sounded great, but then what?

Sharon is a tough lady. She would never retire or slow down. She had two auto accidents last year. Her words of wisdom are profound. She told me, "You just need to move forward with what you're given. There is one thing about a mess. It doesn't move. It will be there when you return. Life is tough. Deal with it and don't complain. You can't retire from life or its problems. If you quit your job, new stresses and problems will take their place. Retiring from a job doesn't mean retiring from life. In fact, going to work helps alleviate a lot of stress and problems. Besides that, you get a paycheck."

Everett is 81. He quipped, "I am still kicking, but I ain't raising the dust I used to."

I see some of Everett in myself. We still try to work as hard as ever, but we just don't have the same capacity and strength we once did.

Ralph is 76. He laughed and told me, "The harder I work, the better I feel. If I don't work, I get plugged up like my carburetor."

Richard is a trucker at age 80. He told me, "I still have the spark; I just don't have the voltage."

Bob, age 85, said, "As long as God lets me do things well,

I'll keep doing them."

Allen, age 82, told me, "The day I sit down, that's the day you can forget me."

Paul is age 86. When I asked him if I would see him next year, he quipped, "If I'm still here, I'll be back."

These men all continue the same theme. "I just don't have the horsepower, but the engine is still going for now."

Vince is 88 and still outspoken. When I asked him about the former president, he grinned and chuckled, "At least other presidents keep their mouths shut so we don't know how dumb they really are."

All these men and women are humorous and profound at the same time. Most of their responses are straightforward, self-deprecating, and have a deeper meaning. They seem to be saying that they know their time on this earth is limited. "So why change now? I've worked hard, so why slow down until they put me in the ground? Why change who I am just because I'm old?" They point out that we probably better just keep doing what we've been doing all our lives and be thankful for each day.

Bennett is a 94-year-old doctor. He worked in the emergency room well into his eighties. He worked with insurance companies until age 93. He planned his retirement for years and finally got around to some version of it at age 94. He walks 150 yards three times a day. He plays bridge every week. He plays in the afternoon because his vision is better then. He also likes to swim.

Bennett is saying that when he slowed down with one job, he had other interests that were nurtured and practiced before he retired. He anticipated what was coming up next and just changed the name of the game, so to speak.

Steve is 82 years old. He runs a bulldozer 4-6 hours a day. He quips, "I used to do it 12 hours a day." He walks on his treadmill 30 minutes each day at a 2.5% grade. He walks his dog every day. He tells me, "I'm not afraid to die. I don't want to lie in bed. Don't want no chemicals in my body! Why prolong dying when the time comes and make my family suffer? You're just alive, and that's all." He reads his Bible every day in the morning and never misses church. He recently went on a mission trip and loved it. This is a man who had a coronary bypass operation and has survived both prostate cancer and malignant melanoma. This is one tough man with strong family ties and deep spiritual beliefs. He lives what he believes. When the time comes, he is saying, "Lord, take me home. I don't want to linger and gripe and be a burden." I think the phrase, "I want to live until I die," applies to Steve. Don't hold back. Take reasonable risks. Persist. Believe. Don't quietly fade into the background. "Retire? Why retire? I'll keep doing what I do until my trip comes to an end."

Several studies have shown associations between believers who attend religious services and living longer lives. One of the most comprehensive, published in JAMA Internal Medicine in 2016, found that women who went to any kind of religious service more than once a week had a 33% lower chance than their secular peers of dying during the 16-year study-follow-up period. Another study found that regular service attendance was linked to reductions in the body's stress responses and even in mortality—so much so that worshippers were 55% less likely to die during the 18-year follow-up period. Factors related to churchgoing–such as having a network of social support, an optimistic attitude, better self-control, and a sense of purpose in life–may account for some long-life benefits in this study and others.[26] Belief in God also provides an intimate spiritual aspect to people's connection to One higher than humans. Believers and frequent churchgoers live up to six or more years longer than their secular counterparts.[27]

Cecil is 84 years old. He has a little store and tries to put in at least 8 hours a day. He says he doesn't sleep well but refuses to consider taking a nap. Unfortunately, he is beginning to lose weight, and that's not a good sign. He tells me, "I just can't seem to do much. I just wear out." He then says, "If I retired, I'd be dead in 30 days."

In his mind and heart, Cecil wants to keep going, but his body is worn out. That's the ultimate fate for all of us. But he also seems to be saying, "maybe I can't do as much, but I can still give the same effort, even though the result isn't the same." Once again, he is telling us not to groan and moan and pine for "the good old days." I think Cecil would just like to go to sleep and not wake up one day. Until that day comes, keep going, realize we aren't guaranteed another day and don't quit. Each day we are blessed to have that day. Keep it up, Cecil!

Glenn is 88 years old. He is very opinionated and loves to tell you what he thinks, even if you don't ask. One of his quips was very disparaging toward former President Trump.

That pretty well summarizes how Glenn approaches life. He has no plans of slowing down or keeping quiet. He is driven by staying relevant and outspoken. I think this gives him the energy to get through the day. He and his mind are active and quick to respond. He has no plans to be quiet and just fade away. As the citizens of our country get older, we need to remember this and continue to make our voices heard. I admit that I admire Glenn's defiance. He reminds us of the privilege we have to express our opinions and defend those whose opinions we may find disagreeable. I'm sure Glenn did not vote for Donald Trump in 2020, but I'm sure he made his vote count.

Stuart is 68 years old. He is a farmer. He still farms 1,000 acres. When I posed the question to him about retiring, he told me, "The American farmer never retires." He chuckled and told me he may "cut back," but not right now. He loves old classic cars. He says he has eight classic "non-rusted" cars that he has restored. He is busy and loves it. He says he may get rid of high-risk activities, but then he grins.

He has the right approach. If you retire from work, whatever that means, something needs to take its place. The transition is easier if you don't completely stop one activity but transition gradually into something else. Stuart is doing this. I'm sure if he really does "cut back" in farming, he will probably "ramp up" his classic car restoration. In short, he won't retire but just change jobs.

Curtis is 65 years old. He told me he likes his work. He was very adamant that he did not want to retire. He plays golf, but not because he really likes golf. He plays golf so he can be with his friends. He admits he doesn't have any hobbies because he has work to fill up his time, so it's never been an issue. He laughed and said he wouldn't want to retire and move to Arizona and sit in the sun. Anyway, it's too hot, he mused. He likes his work, and he likes "to work."

For Curtis, the idea of moving to Arizona means becoming inconsequential and doing what we say we look forward to doing but really dread. The closer we get to the end of our lives, we realize the value of what we have and don't want to lose. Today is pretty good. It is predictable. Tomorrow can be scary, especially if we can't reverse course and get back in the game. We all tend to romanticize "free time" and "sleeping in" until the reality of those thoughts closes in. It seems Curtis has made the right decision to keep working and leave the sands of Arizona to those who already live there and see it as their daily reality.

Devon is a lawyer. He is a very serious man who always seems anxious about something. He never relaxes; he's always thinking. He says he likes his job and his work. He says if he retired, he would no longer be significant, and he would be even more anxious. He travels with his wife but is glad when the trip is over and he can get back to work. He is the owner of his business and tells me he can leave work at four every afternoon if he wants, but he never does and probably never will. He walks three miles at a time, four times a week, to stay fit and relieve stress. Being serious but anxious at the same time is a tough combination on the body and the mind. There is no place to hide. Devon should not retire. It would only increase his anxiety. Devon is like a lot of guys, sort of stuck in life. No real viable plan to replace work. I told him he is relevant; people count on him. Being anxious is often a signal to keep working, take a walk, don't think so much.

Leo is 83 years old. When I asked him about retirement, he told me, "It's like losing your best friend. It's sad that all those things I learned for 46 years I won't use again."

He's right. We invest most of our waking hours learning and doing what we've learned. If we retire, it's all gone. The retirement party ends; then what? Can we become a "new person?" I don't think so. We can get out of bed later, read the newspaper more thoroughly, go for a walk, or volunteer, but all that may quickly get monotonous. Most men and women tell me the same thing. They need a "reason to get up." Weekends are nice, but not seven days a week. All those things we have learned on our journey through life can become insignificant overnight. Traveling always sounds good, but most of us can't wait to get back home. Work is that way. It's nice to have a day off occasionally. We can watch T.V., take a nap, read a book, and visit friends, but at the end of the day, is that enough? Doing that every day may not be so fulfilling.

Preston is 70 years old. He is a lawyer who retired. He talked with one of his colleagues about his own retirement. Preston is not retired anymore. He now stocks shelves at a grocery store and feels calm and fulfilled. When I asked him why he went back to work, he told me, "Well, my two best friends both retired. They're both dead."

He's saying two things. First, he is lonely and needs interaction with others in a work setting. Second, "I better not just sit around." Two sides of the same coin—relationships and doing something to keep busy and engaged. We all do this every day. We complain about our jobs, the weather, the kids, the news, and how the world "should" work. Then when we retire, we may lose our voice, our purpose. Nobody cares what we think. Preston is saying this: If I don't have a job or my friends, what am I supposed to do? If I stock shelves, then I must get up at a certain time and do something that contributes. Hopefully, I can make new "best" friends. Notice he's saying, "I don't have to be a lawyer, but I do need to work." He'll probably keep stocking shelves for several years.

William is 70. He has lung cancer but still smokes cigarettes. He also has a specialized pacemaker for his heart, but his emotional heart isn't doing well. "They told me at work they wouldn't force me to retire, but they also said they didn't have any work for me to do," he said. Sounds like forced retirement to me. Then he said his day now consisted of lying in bed, going to the bathroom, and watching T.V. He doesn't have family or friends to help him through the transition.

William "needs" to work. It defined his life. He didn't plan for retirement or being told, "we don't have any work for you to do." I told him to go back and find another job. There are many places that could use his experience and desire to contribute. He also might feel better if he gave up or cut back on the cigarettes.

Jeffrey is 84 and has many different medical problems. He told me that thirteen of his friends retired, and only three are still alive. He continues to farm full time, and bales hay— very hard, physical labor. He takes care of twenty-six horses by himself. He lamented, "We don't have any mushrooms this year." Mushroom hunters abound in the area, tromping through woodlands in search of the morels.

He is certainly a man who should continue to work. He sounds like a guy who wants to live life fully until his time on the Earth ends. I tell him I'll see him in the office next year. He plans on it as well.

There are so many aspects to retirement. One is the drastic change in daily physical and mental activity. If we don't have to get up at five every morning, do we now sleep in until nine? Do we go to bed at eleven every night instead of nine? If there is no schedule and timetable to dictate our daily activities, do we become overweight, lazy, and cynical? Not necessarily, nor does it seem very desirable.

If you do decide to retire, you need to make a plan ahead of time to keep your mind and body fit. It will take work, but it must be done. Then refine the plan as you go along.

Read every day.

Work to keep the mind sharp—do puzzles of any sort, crosswords, sudoku, play bridge; do whatever you enjoy and challenges the mind.

Get hold of an old math book and do algebra or calculus problems.

Brush up on the foreign language you studied in high school.

Volunteer at an organization that interests you and where you can contribute. Don't underestimate your well-earned years of wisdom.

Stay involved.

Catch up with old friends. Make new friends.

Don't slow down.

Exercise every day for at least thirty minutes.

Take a walk or ride a bike. It doesn't need to be fancy.

Take a nap.

Eat reasonable day-to-day nutritious meals that you can keep up forever. Don't diet—all diets end.

Limit the snacks.

Don't try to fill the boredom with alcohol consumption.

Get enough sleep.

Be consistent.

All of this seems simple yet hard to do and maintain.

Some of my patients have told me they've lost a sense of worth or purpose, and regret having retired. I tell them that every time that thought occurs, go out and take a walk, literally. Anxiety, anger, and remorse improve when we exercise our minds and bodies. Disappointment is one of the five emotional stages of retirement, including planning for retirement, excitement about retirement, building a new purpose in life, and finally, routine and stability.[28]

There's a lot of information about retirement from financial advisors and on the internet, but not as much regarding retirement decisions outside the financial ones. People need to know how to plan for filling their time and changing their perspectives. Planning for a new way of life ahead, both financially and emotionally, and adapting the plan as time goes on are key factors in a satisfying and fulfilling life in retirement.

The definition of "work" has changed a great deal in our lifetimes with the advent of the digital age. Various kinds of "work" can be done from home, without requiring a physical presence at the office. Meetings among colleagues around the world are done virtually. Even medical visits are sometimes done virtually. Admittedly, working online is very different from physically taxing hard labor, such as construction work, working in a grocery store, or being a hard-working nurse.

There are now roughly 77 million "Baby Boomers" in our country. They carry an average credit card balance of $6,747 and $25,812 in total non-mortgage debt. They have a 3.2% delinquency rate for accounts 90 to 180 days past due. Boomer homeowners carry an average mortgage debt of $191,650.29.[29] They hold more than five times the borrowing obligations Americans their age held two decades ago—the first time in history that such a high degree of debt has been seen so late in life. Debt in the past peaked for people in their 40s. Median savings for U.S. households nearest retirement age dropped 32% between 2007 and 2017 to $14,500. The net worth of Americans aged 55-64 is lower than the same age group surveyed in 1989.[30] *They can't retire!* In February 2019, about 20% of Americans over 65 were either working or looking for work.[31] Something doesn't make sense. We are living longer but not being very intelligent about how we manage those extra years.

The coronavirus pandemic has accentuated financial angst about Americans' retirement plans. More than half, 51%, say that the pandemic has increased concerns about achieving financial security in retirement. Although the nation is highly polarized on many things, Americans are united in their worry about retirement issues.[32]

The recent doubling of gasoline prices and food price increases place the burden of financial insecurity at the forefront of our minds when we think about whether to retire. Thus, we are living longer, spending more, and something must change. It may take us a few years as a nation to get it right. Hopefully, we will look back on the pandemic as a learning situation and gain a new perspective on many areas of life and retirement.

Maybe we shouldn't retire!

My Thoughts and Perspective

When people lived to age 40, decisions about retirement had no relevance. But through the 20th century came Social Security, Medicare, better health care, and better working conditions, resulting in longer lives. The fact of the matter is that even in the 1970s, men only lived to about age 70. Now grouchy old men live to 75 or 80, and women live more than 80 years on average. As a result, the question of "what to do" in old age suddenly became an issue. Some people keeping to themselves, just faded away, and one day, "Grandpa passed away." Then came the concept of retirement communities for those with the means to afford to live out their lives there. Some who live in these communities have remarked to me that they are bored. They play bingo, watch T.V., and eat too much. They want to go back to the "bad old days." They think, "If I drift off in obscurity, spending all I have, then what have I left in monetary assets to pass on to my children?"

Some tell me that after they retired, no one asked what their opinions were on current issues. This further isolates and devalues the retiree. "I guess we don't count anymore," I was told by one patient.

"Why should I take my medications?"

"Why should I follow a diet?"

"Who cares?"

Often the response I hear is, "I will not take my meds." Then I remind them that people do care about them. Families want their wisdom. Grandkids need their stories—tell them about the "good old days."

"Life was better then."

"The world is going to hell."

"When I was young, my dad never let me get away with that!"

The problem is that, as a society, we are getting old. Too many medical tests are done on too many people. "If it ain't broke, don't fix it" is a better approach. All of this is made more evident if we retire. In a sense, we lose control of our destiny. Often decisions are made for us rather than by us. Daily activities become more challenging as time goes on.

The silence and the isolation in retirement can be the

worst for some people. Add to that the effects of the Covid-19 pandemic and rising inflation. Rates of mental illness, depression, and suicide have increased throughout all age groups and across professions. Psychological and social impacts have been profound and will persist.

With so many people currently working from home, even the definition of work and retirement are changing, and the distinction between them can become blurred. "If I don't bring home a paycheck, what is my value?"

It all reflects on our work, defining who we are. Many of us have worked hard all our lives and equate our worth with our jobs and what we produce. It's probably not a good view of ourselves, but it's often true. Do you see any prime-time ads on television catering to the elderly besides arthritis and gastrointestinal medications? Hearing aids, Medicare supplements, walk-in tubs, and stairlifts are marketed to this group.

This book is not intended to be a condemnation of moving forward with retirement. If you do want to retire, though, you need to make a plan that begins on Day One of your new life in retirement. It will need to be realistic and flexible and change as life changes. Retirement defines a "new you," but you will still be the same person when it comes to your value system, family, friends, and fundamental day-to-day issues.

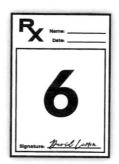

Have I Saved Enough?

First, retirement means no steady, reliable work-related income. Ask yourself, have I really saved enough? Do I have enough to cover ongoing debt? Do I need to change my investment strategy from trying to make an extra dollar to preserving what I have? What kind of risk can I tolerate? How much Social Security will I receive? Are the kids finished with their education? Do I help with their mortgage? And so it goes…

I don't ever want to be a burden to my family. How do I make sure that doesn't happen? What am I going to do to keep busy? I want to do "meaningful" things. Do I volunteer? Do I find another type of part-time job? Where? How do I find out? Should I develop a hobby? Should I be worried about how I spend my final days? How do I want to be remembered?

It sounds morbid to me, but now may be the best time to discuss these issues with family and friends.

Do I set limits on my care now as I anticipate my life on Earth nearing its end in the future? Should I? Does the family want me to do that? Most of all, I want my wife to be taken care of no matter what.

What a mess! We start reading the obituaries looking for friends. We relive our younger "glory days," our successes, and our failures. "If I die, what will my obituary say?"

Work is good in so many ways. It keeps us in the present and helps us plan for the future. It keeps us connected, optimistic, and alive.

So, I ask you, *do you really want to retire?*

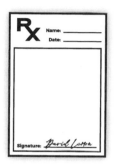

Epilogue

I wrote the following in 2007:

I believe that every day is another chance to set things right.

I believe that people are inherently good, not evil, and that given the right incentives and opportunities, we all want to do the right thing, whatever that means.

I am a doctor, and this belief nags at me to listen more intently and act more decisively, but also to worry more intensely about how my family and patients will cope.

I grew up watching *Father Knows Best* and hearing General Electric tell me that "Progress is our most important product." I believed that then. I still do. I have changed my opinion about what progress *really* means. I don't think it means more and newer iPhones, but I'm still working on that one.

My beliefs have been challenged repeatedly during my personal and professional life. My parents were killed in an airplane crash almost three decades ago. I was lost for many years after that. I felt cheated. Their approval was important to me. I worked for twelve years to become a cardiologist, and then my parents, whose blessing I needed, were gone. Gradually, however, I have come to appreciate who they were and, as a result, who I am. My father was also a doctor. I see some of his patients now, thirty years later. They remember him. They see me, and in seeing me, maybe they see him. It is comforting to them to see continuity and the passing of the torch.

I often visit my parents' gravesite. It is rather inconspicuous, but the inscription reads, "Ken and Marge Lemon, Two Good People." I think that pretty well says it all.

At age 60, I'm sure I'm closer to the end than the beginning, but I relish every step of the way. I still love my work and the people, and yes, trying to help them. When they recount to me that I took care of their mother twenty years ago, and she is just fine, I usually smile and say, "I guess I must have done something right." What greater gift can they give me? You see, that is enough. It's what makes me want to keep doing what I do. I am blessed. *This*, I believe.

Here I am now, fifteen years later, in 2022, writing this and still at it. I still think the work I do is valuable. In the last fifteen years since writing the above, I have lost my son, my brother, my sister, and a beloved dog. I have a beautiful, talented wife, three wonderful new grandchildren, and one dog. I am thankful for them each day. And I still don't want to retire.

I am blessed!

Endnotes

1. https://www.theatlantic.com/business/archive/2014/10/how-retirement-was-invented/381802

2. https://www.theatlantic.com/business/archive/2014/10/how-retirement-was-invented/381802

3. https://www.reuters.com/article/us-japan-economy-retirement-idUSKCN1RM0GP

4. https://take-profit.org/en/statistics/retirement-age-men/france/

5. https://www.pewresearch.org/fact-tank/2019/01/17/where-millennials-end-and-generation-z-begins/

6. https://www.cdc.gov/healthcommunication/pdf/
    audience/audienceinsight_boomers.pdf

7. https://www.wsj.com/articles/people-are-going-out-
    again-but-not-to-the-office-11644843600

8. https://www.bu.edu/articles/2021/alcohol-consumption-
    has-spiked-during-the-pandemic-could-the-
    consequences-outlast-coronavirus/

9. https://www.nextavenue.org/retirement-alcohol-abuse/

10. https://www.pewresearch.org/fact-tank/2020/11/09/
    the-pace-of-boomer-retirements-has-accelerated-in-
    the-past-year/#:~:text=In%20the%20third%20quarter
    %20of,the%20same%20quarter%20of%202019

11. https://www.brookings.edu/research/covid-19-and-
    retirement-impact-and-policy-responses/

12. https://www.investmentnews.com/covid-19-causing-
    retirees-postpone-retirement-202486

13. https://www.nirsonline.org/wpcontent/uploads/2021/02/
    FINAL-Retirement-Insecurity-2021-.pdf

14. https://www.cnbc.com/2022/05/31/25percent-of-
    americans-are-delaying-retirement-due-to-
    inflation.html

15. https://pubmed.ncbi.nlm.nih.gov/33562869/

16. https://www.health.harvard.edu/staying-healthy/exercise-and-aging-can-you-walk-away-from-father-time

17. https://www.cdc.gov/nchs/pressroom/nchs_press_releases/2021/202107.htm

18. https://magazine.jhsph.edu/2020/covid-19-and-suicide-crisis-within-crisis

19. https://hrsonline.isr.umich.edu

20. https://www.health.harvard.edu/blog/is-retirement-good-for-health-or-bad-for-it-201212105625

21. https://www.aier.org/article/the-collapse-of-trust-in-public-health

22. https://www.nextavenue.org/retirement-life-women-and-men-do-it-very-differently

23. https://www.azquotes.com/quotes/topics/attitude.html

24. https://aging.com/how-to-cope-with-the-aging-process

25. https://www.health.harvard.edu/staying-healthy/exercise-and-aging-can-you-walk-away-from-father-time

26. https://time.com/5159848/do-religious-people-live-longer

27. https://www.sciencedaily.com/releases/1999/05/
990517064323.htm

28. https://saveinvestandretire.com/get-ready-for-5-most-
common-emotional-stages-of-retirement

29. https://www.cnbc.com/select/how-much-debt-do-baby-
boomers-have

30. https://on.wsj.com/3CiMAc9

31. https://www.businessinsider.com/personal-
finance/baby-boomers-working-past-retirement-age-
healthier-2019-4?op=1

32. https://www.nirsonline.org/reports/
retirementinsecurity2021